TAI JI

Essential Tai Ji

by
Chungliang Al Huang

with photographs by
Si Chi Ko

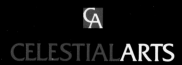

CELESTIALARTS

Copyright © 2001, 1989
  Chungliang Al Huang

CELESTIAL ARTS
P.O. Box 7123
Berkeley, CA 94707
www.tenspeed.com

Distributed in Australia by Simon and
Schuster Australia, in Canada by Ten Speed
Press Canada, in New Zealand by Southern
Publishers Group, in South Africa by Real
Books, in Southeast Asia by Berkeley Books,
and in the United Kingdom and Europe by
Airlift Books.

Photographs © Si Chi Ko
Cover design by Betsy Stromberg
Edited by Suzanne Pierce

Library of Congress Cataloging-in-Publication
Data on file with the publisher.

This edition ISBN: 1-58761-109-0
First Celestial Arts ISBN:
  1-89087-556-1

First American Printing, 1989
1 2 3 4 5 6 7 8 9 10 —
  05 04 03 02 01

Printed in Hong Kong

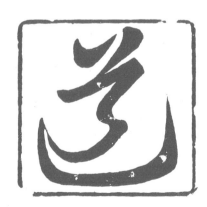

Contents

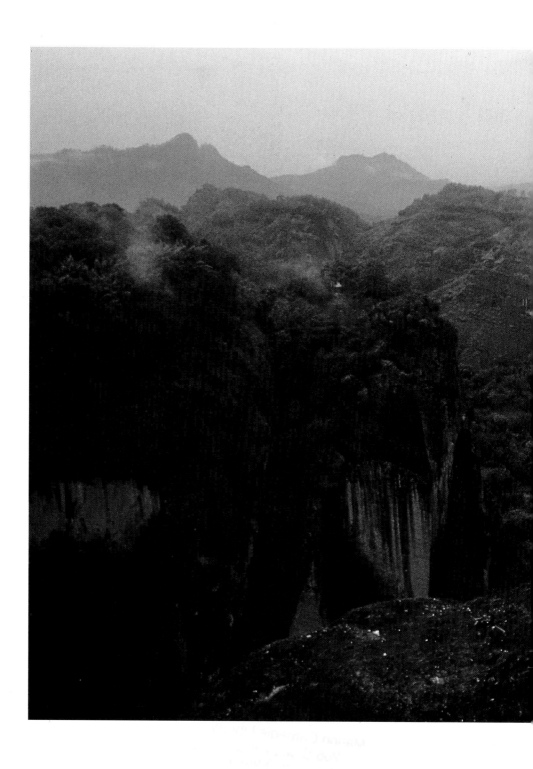

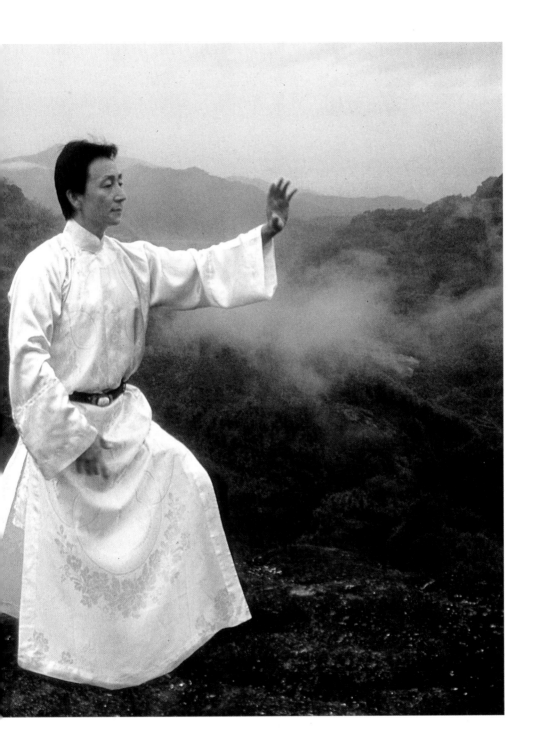

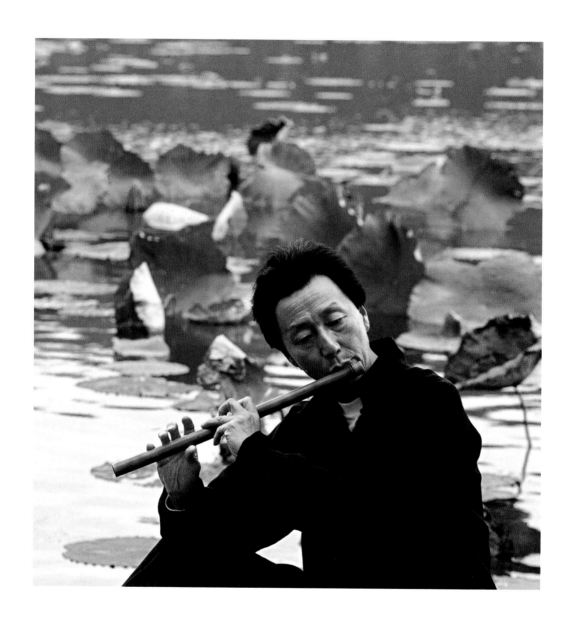

I   Introduction

Tai Ji is a universal medium for the cultivation of Body, Mind and Spirit.

It is natural. It is perennial. It is for everyone, of all ages.

It is easy to learn. It can be joyful and exciting to practice.

It is a dance of life to be treasured.

It is for you.

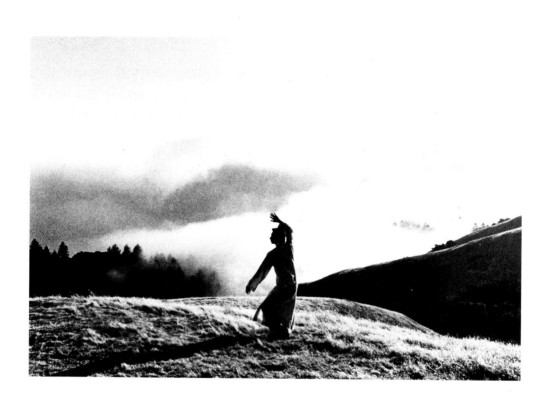

II The Origin of Tai Ji

Tai Ji Myths

Fu Hsi, the mythical ruler of China's first dynasty, Hsia (2205–1766 B.C.), invented the Tai Ji practice, and his revelations about the transformation of the universe became the original diagrams of the ancient book, the *I Ching*.

A Taoist monk, probably during Tang Dynasty (618–906 A.D.), was inspired to create Tai Ji while observing a combat between a snake and a sparrow.

Another monk, in Yuan Dynasty (1279–1368 A.D.), learned to do Tai Ji in a dream.

Other stories—historically more factual—are about recluses throughout the ages who created Tai Ji as healthful meditations, and for self-defense purposes.

But my favorite story is the next one. . . .

The Real Fairytale

Once upon a time, somewhere, anywhere in the world, there was a man (or a woman) sitting on a mountain top, quietly observing nature. He became so inspired by the movements of the world around him that he began to dance, imitating all the natural elements he could easily identify. He opened himself completely to the forces of nature. He became the forces: sky, earth, fire, water, trees, flowers, wind, cloud, birds, fishes and butterflies. His dance became ecstatic, completely transforming and transcendent. So happy with himself, he then poetically named each movement motif: Bubble of the Cosmos, Yin/Yang Harmonic Loop, White Cranes Flashing Wings, Cloud-Waving Hands, Golden Birds Balancing on One Leg, Embrace Tiger Return to Mountain.

He or she was the originator of the Tai Ji dance. His moment of creation could have happened thousands of years ago or could have happened right now, this moment, somewhere, anywhere in the world. This person could be you.

You are the potential Tai Ji creator. You are the dancer and the dance.

ENJOY!

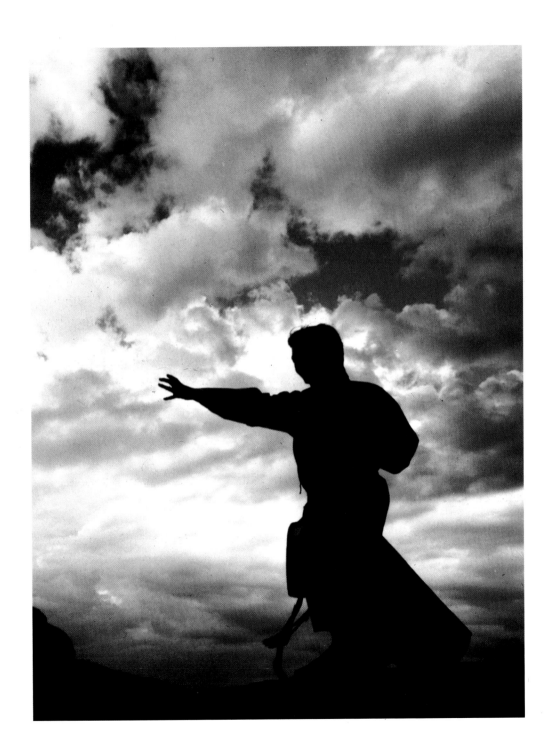

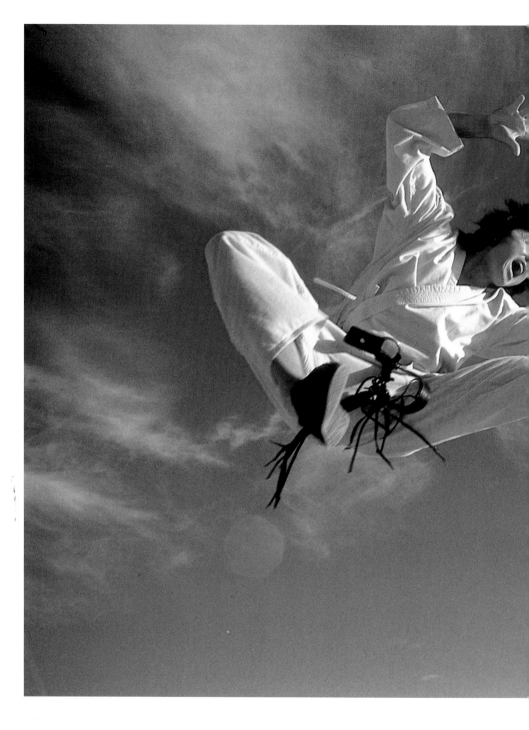

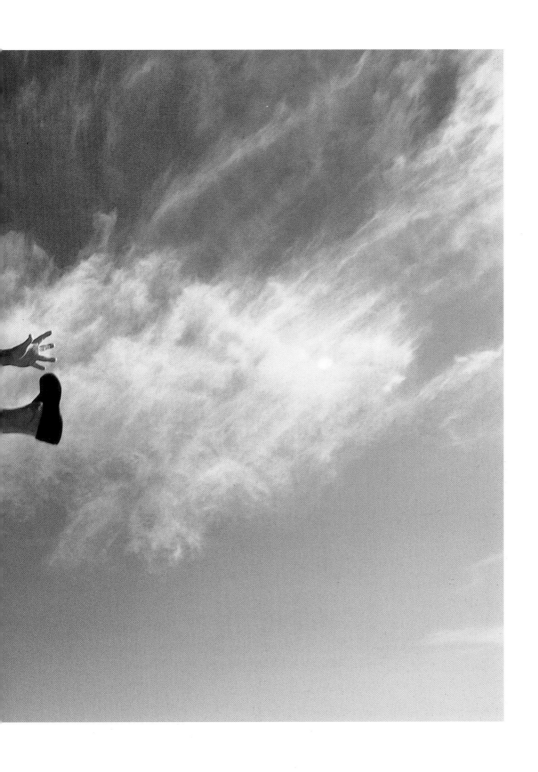

Observe the written Chinese characters of Tai and Ji:

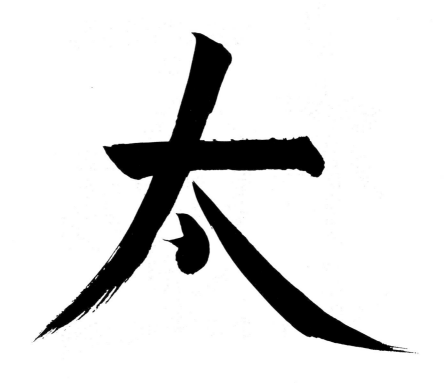

TAI
The word Tai looks like
a wide open human body concentrating on
the potential lifeforce within.

III The Meaning of Tai Ji

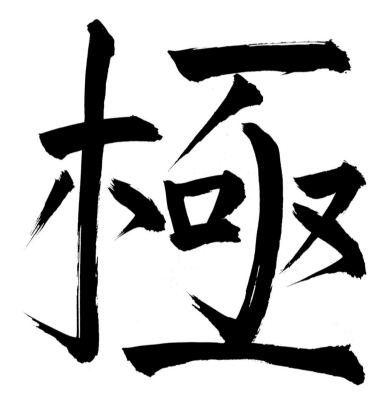

JI
The Word Ji is an elaboration
of the continual exploration of this
moving body meditation.

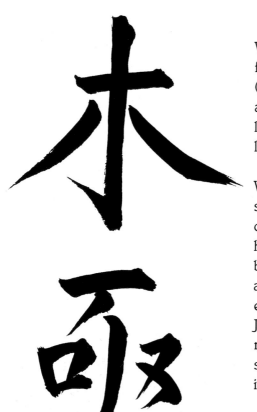

We identify with the growing tree—from root (our feet and legs) to trunk (pelvis and torso), then out to branches and twigs (arms and fingers), to leaves, blossoms and fruits (our endless creative expressions).

We recognize the humble human, stretched within our potential power, connected between heaven (upper horizontal stroke) and earth (lower base stroke) to unify (circle-square) and to interact (figure 8 infinity loop) eternally as we recycle our energies. Ji is a blueprint, a guide, a mirror reflection of our body as teacher. It shows the body's innate intelligence, its wisdom.

Tai Ji literally means the "great ultimate" of practical daily living.

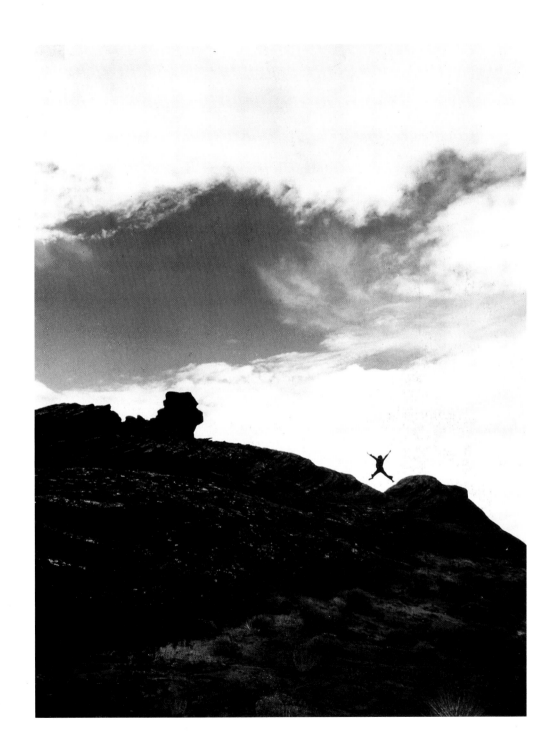

Tai Ji movement, as with nature,
has little to do with
human purposefulness,
ego-control, or
calculating analysis.

It simply IS.

We describe Tai Ji as the
no-mind,
no-control,
no-purpose
Dance of Nature,
of
Living.

If the many legs of a centipede were
controlled by thinking mechanisms,
the poor creature would never take
another step.

IV The Vocabulary of Tai Ji

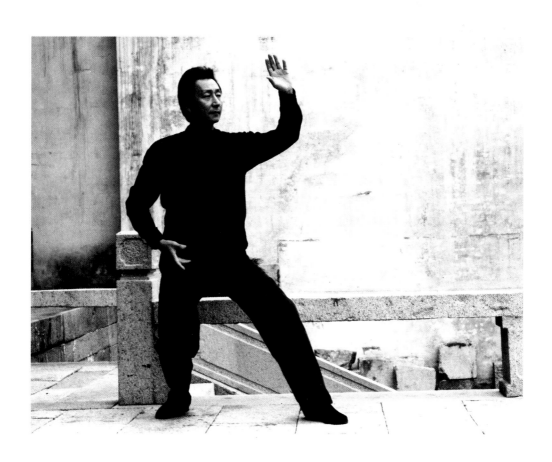

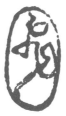

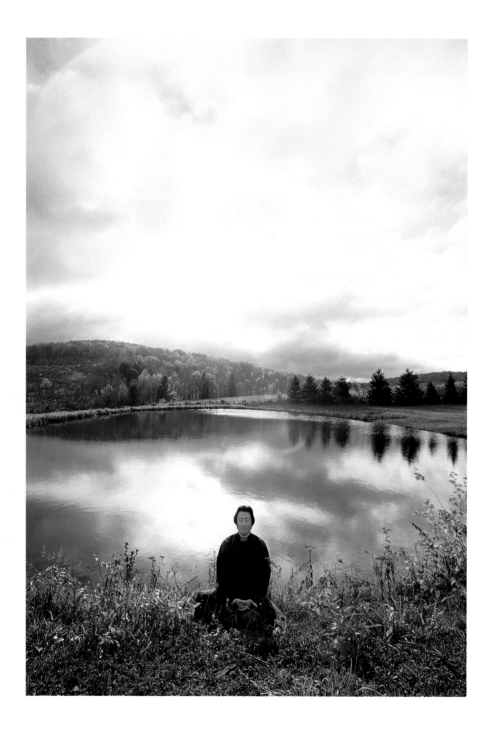

The Concept of Chi

Chi is the forces of the Cosmos, between heaven and earth. It is the primal life energy that we receive from our parents, as they received from their ancestors since the beginning of time.

Chi is the air we breathe, and the food we eat, and the enveloping atmosphere, both natural and unnatural, that we respond to. It is emotional, psychical and attitudinal feelings and sensations, according to our human responses to life.

When we feel good about our environment and the people around us, we feel more energized. We have more Chi power. Tai Ji practice teaches us to enhance this power in our lives by using our bodies effectively, as channels for energy of the lifeforces in our daily activities.

Therefore, some of the most basic exercises for beginners in Tai Ji involve proper breathing and proper body postures through simple movements.

They will become easy and joyful if we understand and remember the meanings and original creativity of their practice.

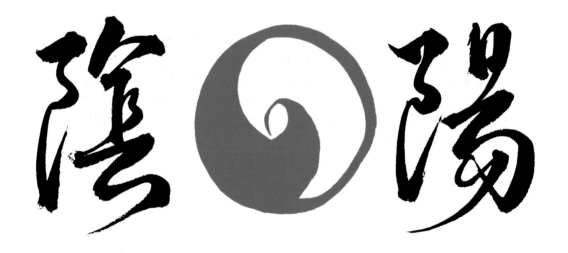

Yin/Yang Polarity

The original meaning shown in the Chinese written characters depicts the ever-changing shady and sunny sides of a mountain. It is a philosophy of continuous interplay of the natural forces, such as night and day alternating, warm and cold seasons changing in cycles, and woman and man coupling and harmonizing. Yin/Yang is a complete concept with dual possibilities, inseparable and constantly striving to complement and unify.

In Tai Ji, every posture and movement is based on transforming duality into Yin/Yang polarity.

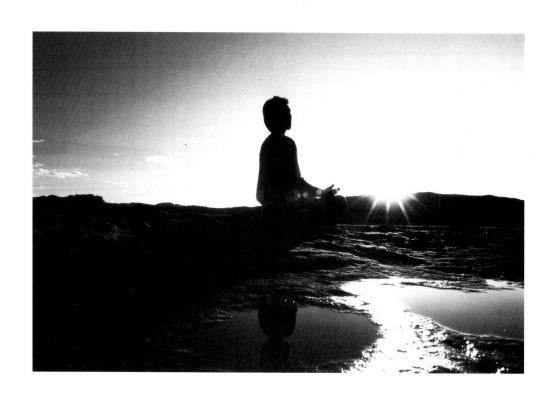

Dantien

The literal meaning of Dantien is the field (or reservoir) of vital essence, the gut force in the belly. It is a centered and contained power-feeling inside and around the lower abdomen.

In Tai Ji, every gesture of the Chi-flow begins and ends in the Dantien.

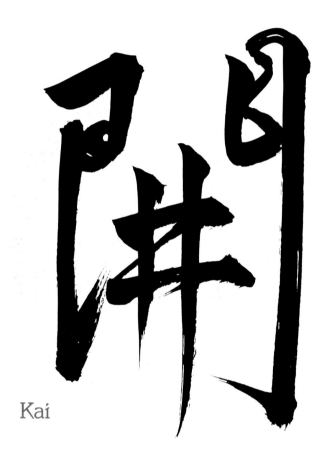

Kai

Kai means to open, expand, unlock and unleash.
It is often used in Yin/Yang polarity to complement
the closing and gathering gestures in Tai Ji.

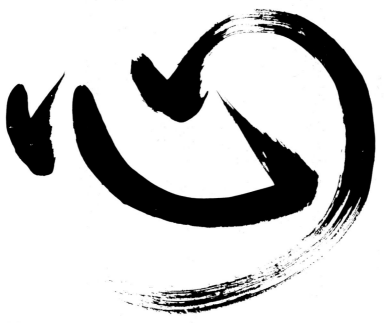

Hsing

In Chinese, Hsing means both the Mind and the Heart,
the unified consciousness of Mind/Body/Spirit.
In Tai Ji, the Heart and Mind (Hsing)
of the human consciousness is focused
in the Dantien.

Take time to become
re-acquainted with
running down the hill,
spreading your arms like wings,
reaching up to the blue sky
on the mountain top, and
extending beyond the horizon
across the sea.

Remember how your body feels
swimming downstream,
effortlessly
being carried away.

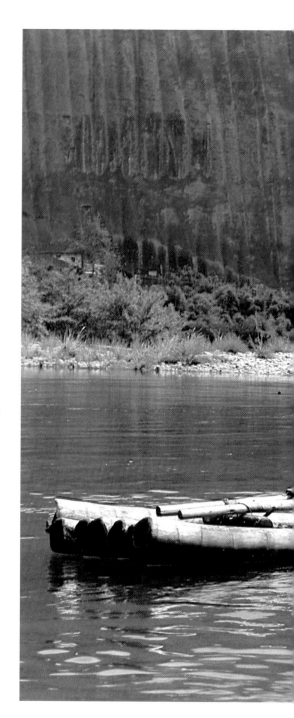

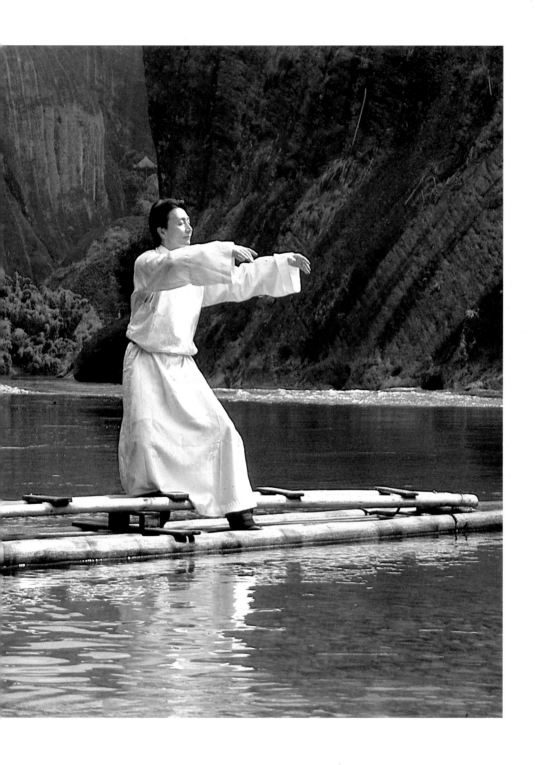

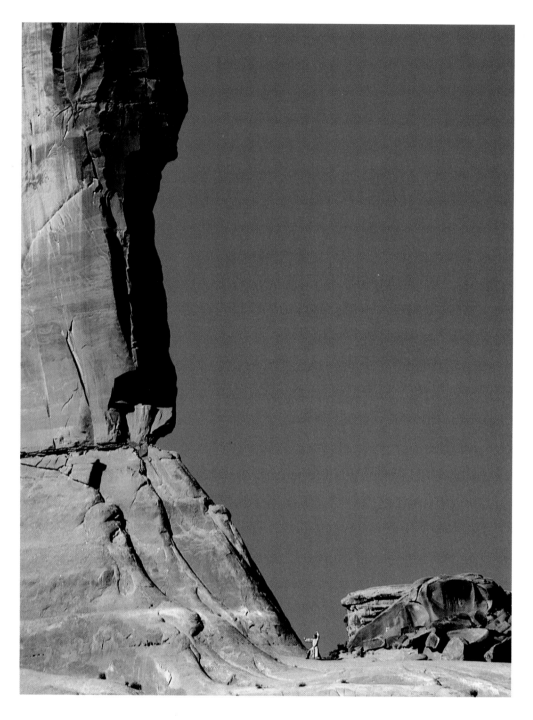

Human being is very small

but

Chi-power is immense

Sky is unlimited

So is Earth.

V The Benefit of Tai Ji

Tai Ji frees the body and helps with relaxation and overall circulation. It activates muscles, sinews and joints in the body. It strengthens physical power without stress.

It maintains youth and aliveness, and slows down the aging process through rejuvenation.

Tai Ji calms and collects. It clears and sharpens the mind to help us in focusing and centering our daily activities.

When the body and mind move harmoniously together, the human spirit soars.

Tai Ji helps to balance the conflict of duality, as mind and body polarize and unite. It reinforces soft approaches to otherwise hard living.

Tai Ji promotes a welcome meeting of the East and the West and reaffirms the importance of global awareness.

Tai Ji for the individual is a microcosm of the world at large. Through our personal experience of Tai Ji, we begin to understand the macrocosm of the universe.

The ultimate benefit of Tai Ji is to experience living in a healthful and wide-awake state of being.

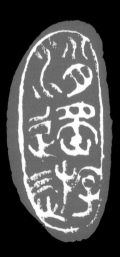

The practice will endure and its benefits will sustain you!

Learn to open yourself.

Stretch your arms. Open your legs. Open your eyes,
your throat.

Breathe.

Open your chest, your gut, your pelvis.
Open your Dantien.

Open your heart and your mind.
Relax and breathe.

You will find your horizons expanding,
your vision improving...

Enjoy this open arm, open-mind,
open-heart position.

Tai Ji is Joy and Happiness.

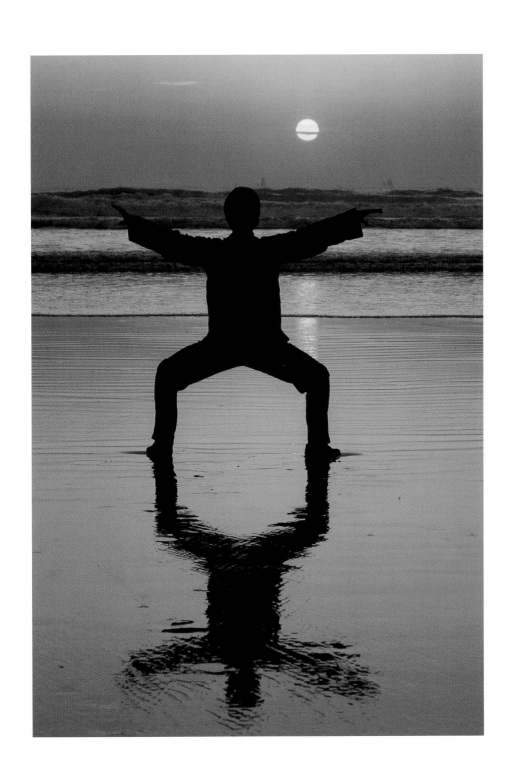

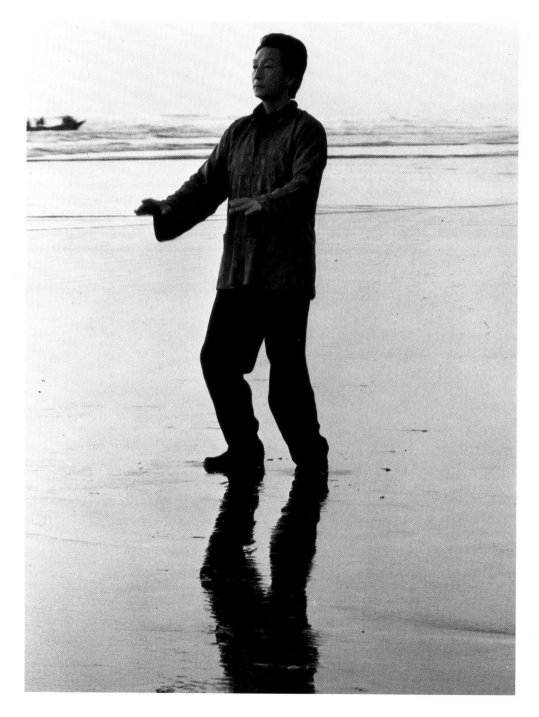

VI The Form of Tai Ji: Some Basic Moves

Tai Ji Stance

Before we begin, it is essential to identify the basic stance used in Tai Ji. Your legs are directly under your pelvis, feet comfortably apart and parallel. Your body is relaxed, with spine erect, as if suspended from the sky.

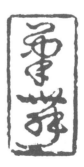

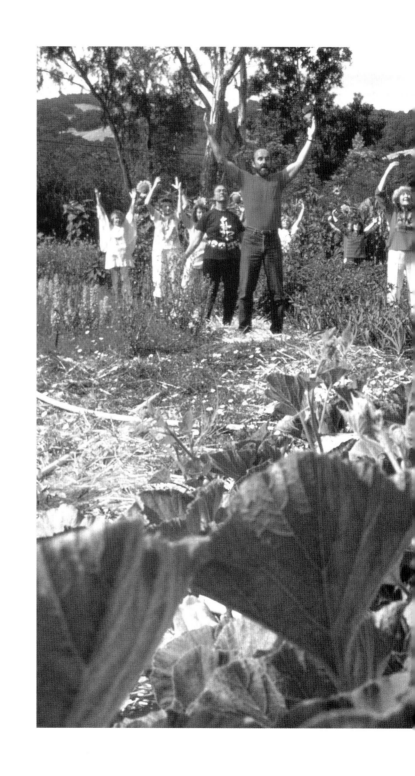

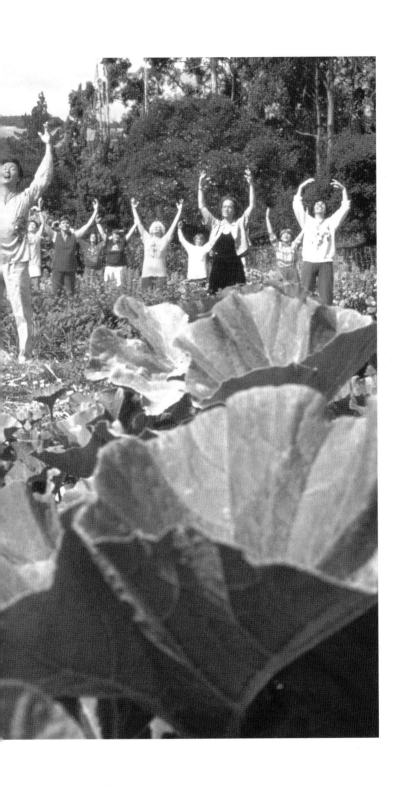

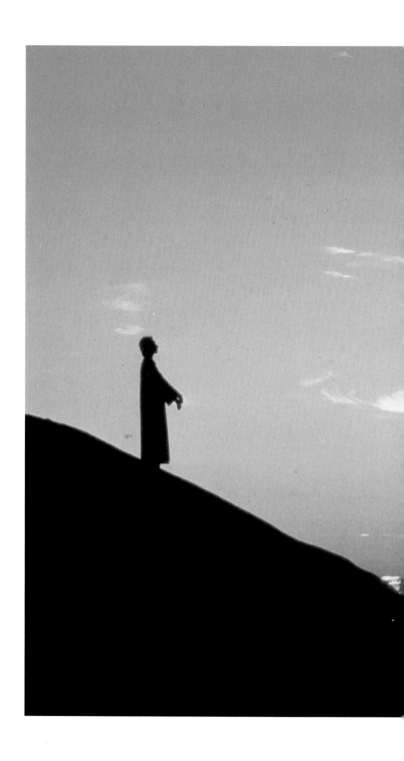

Connect To The Earth

Feel the gravity of the earth pulling you toward its center.

Relax and bend your knees as you explore the energy coming from the earth.

Feel a gentle "digging in" and releasing of your body, like a pump soaking up the Earth-Chi into your Dantien.

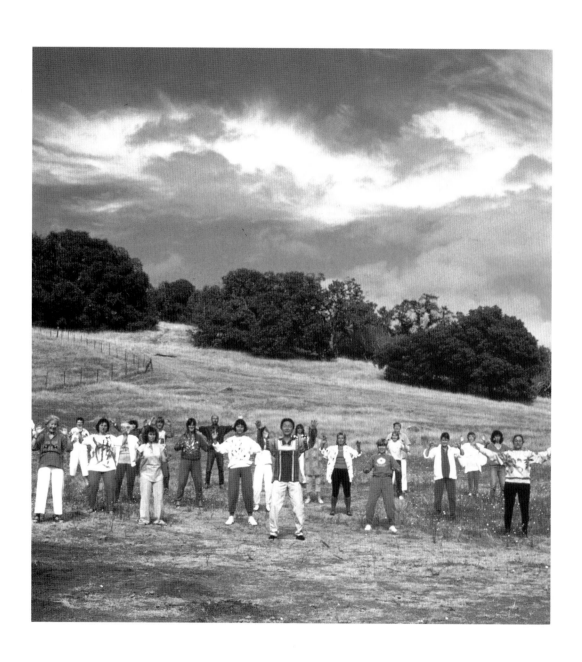

The Earth/Sky Circle

Combine the above Sky and Earth poles into one circular, open-armed movement.

Place your hands on your Dantien. Inhale, and feel your body filling with Earth energy. Let this energy grow upward as your arms rise in front of you until they are above your head.

Open your arms to the sky as you release your breath. Now continue to exhale as your arms float down through the sides. Let them return naturally back to your Dantien.

As you practice, be aware of the inseparable connection between your movement and your breathing. One must induce and respond to the other.

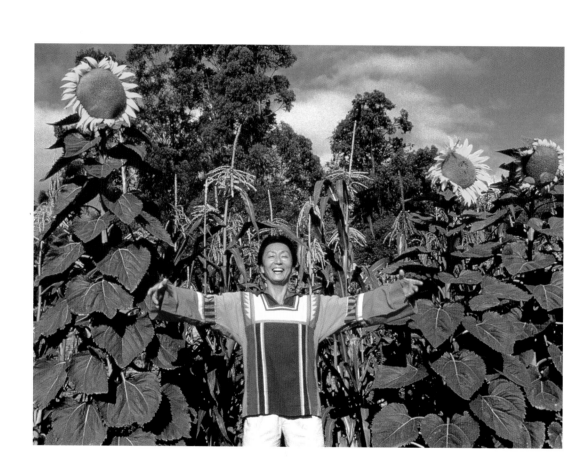

Kai Hsing

Begin in the basic stance. Let your hands cross in front of your upper chest, directly under your throat.

Take a step back, as you push open your arms horizontally to the sides.

Feel centered in this new expanded position.

Now, bring the weight back to the original position, by stepping in and retracting the arms.

As you practice, alternate stepping back with one foot, then the other.

The movement has an expanding, telescopic action that is regulated by your breathing. As you expand your breath, you expand your horizon. As you release your breath, you collect the movement back in.

Feel the movement following the natural open/close, out/in bellow action of the lungs.

This Kai Hsing movement is very important for proper breathing, good balance, and smooth transitions in all weight-shifting motifs of Tai Ji practice.

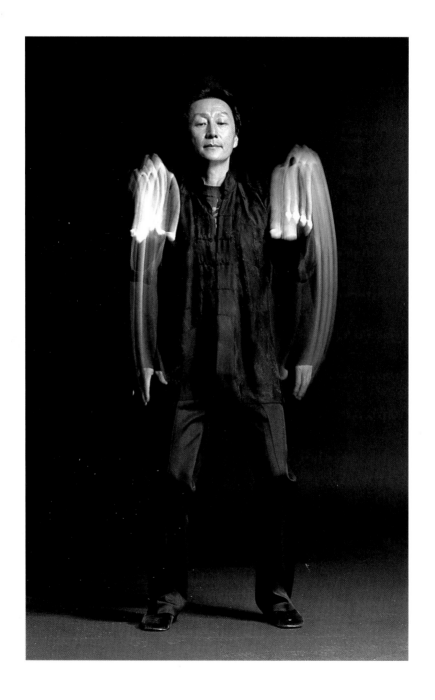

Rise and Fall with Arms

Assume the basic Tai Ji stance. Meditate on your breathing pattern, visualising your Chi flowing from heels to crown of head, circulating through your entire body sequentially and freely.

Slowly inhale and raise the arms forward, until they are extended in front of your chest. Exhale and let the arms float back down to the side.

Keep your body relaxed and resiliant, especially in your knees.

Refrain from dictating the actions with muscles. Instead, imagine the arms light and hollow, as the Chi forces inside and around, and especially underneath, begin to awaken and guide your arms upward.

Be aware of the relaxation of your elbows and wrists. Allow the gravity to support them as the arms glide upward, and downward.

Visualize your energybody extending beyond the physical self. That is, allow the space around you and between your arms and legs to become an expanded and supporting element of your movement.

Notice, particularly, how the space under your floating arms begins to be more tangible and substantial.

As you repeat this rise-return/inhale-exhale movement, allow the length of the body to stretch and collect. Utilize the attraction of the sky above and earth beneath.

You will begin to feel your energy and breathing capacity increase, as you move gently up and down, out and in, like an accordion.

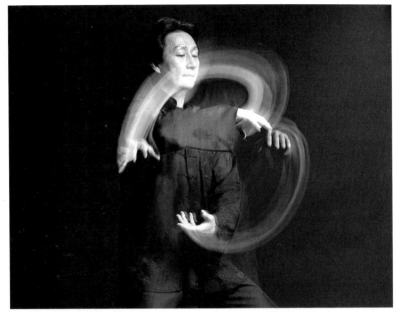

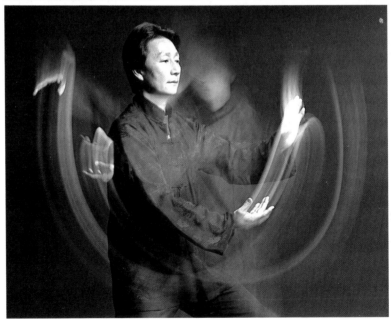

Moving the Yin/Yang Sphere

To feel initial energy, rub your palms vigorously and cup the heat generated within. Form it into a small, warm rotating ball, gently cradled between your hands.

Let it grow to include the elbow, and slowly begin to shape and form the energy into an infinity/Moebius strip-like pattern.

Keeping your spine as a centerpole, expand the sphere to include your shoulders and chest. Then continue to encompass the whole front of your torso.

Finally, you will feel the energy growing to surround your whole body. You will need to pivot, naturally following the movement from side to side.

Your feet, knees and hips must move together, and the spine must continue to act as an upright center.

This revolving sphere of Chi that you now embrace and embody will eventually take you into more complicated moving patterns in Tai Ji.

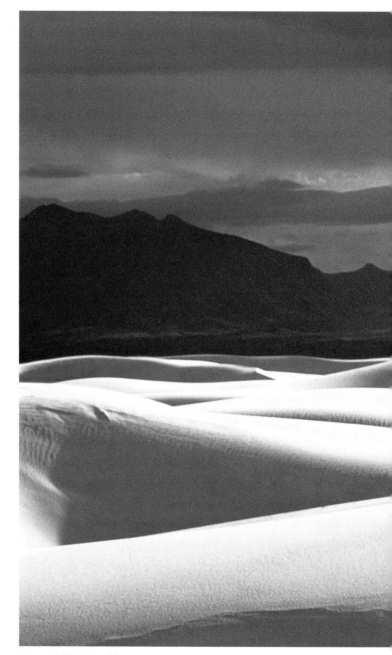

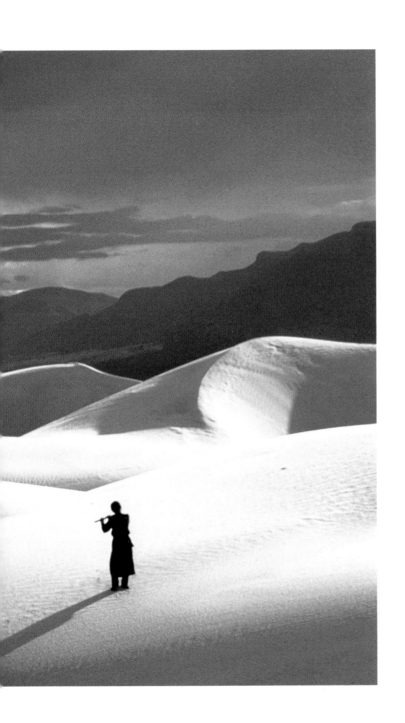

The metaphors of Tai Ji motifs are beautifully evocative.

Their poetic images inspire and guide.

But do not cling to them.

The ancient Chinese sages expressed it this way:

"Use the bridge to cross the great water,
but there is no need to carry the bridge
on your shoulders looking for the next water."

Put even more succinctly:
"After you get the message, hang up the phone!"

In Tai Ji, we try SOFTER!

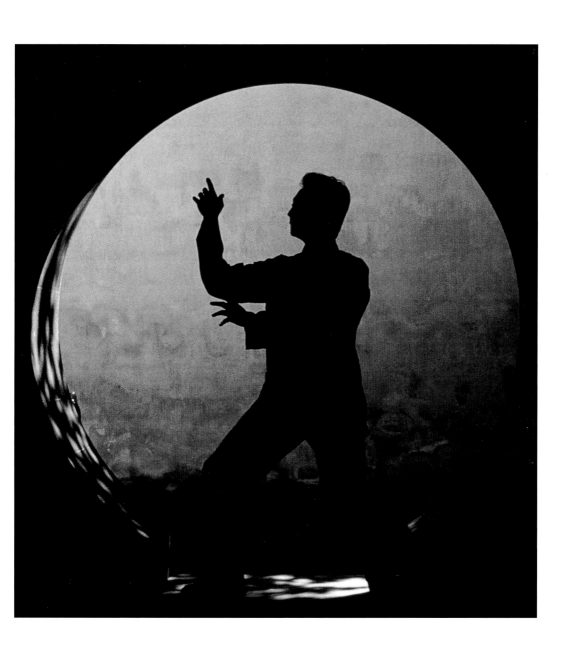

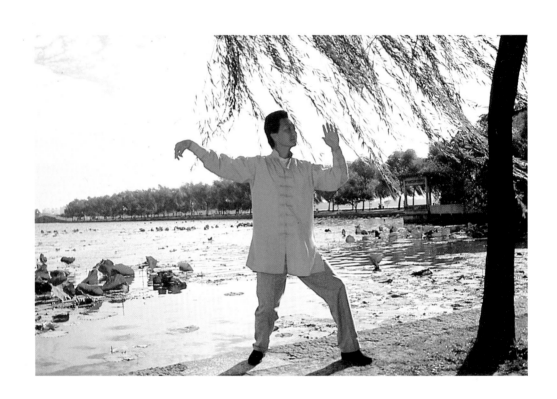

VII The Tai Ji Dance:
The Five Moving Forces

Fire

Wood   **Earth**   Gold

Water

Over the years, I have developed and crystalized an organic choreography of five motifs that has proved to be a gratifying vehicle for early Tai Ji learners. In it, the elemental life forces are used metaphorically to inspire a kinesthetic awareness within our bodies.

You will begin by identifying the Chi-power of the individual metaphors, but will soon learn to connect them in an organically-evolving sequence.

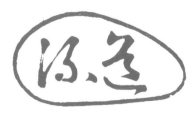

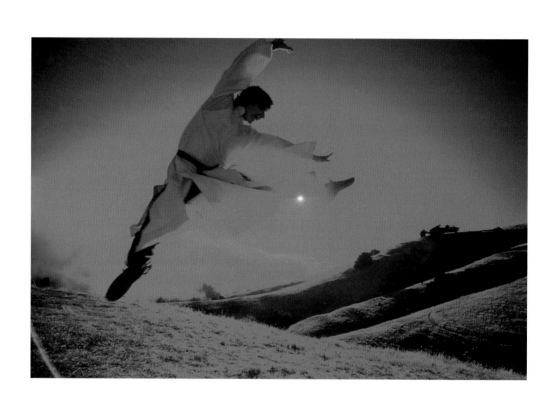

Fire

Fire is the lifeforce you feel from within, ready to be released outward and upward like a flame.

Stand centered. Put both hands in front of the Dantien and begin to stoke up the Chi within, as if the belly were a furnace.

Now send the energy forward, by taking a step and pushing the power out front and up. (In doing so, your feet have shifted to a new position. Always retain the upright and balanced center of weight between both legs. Do not become "lopsided.")

Fire is to give

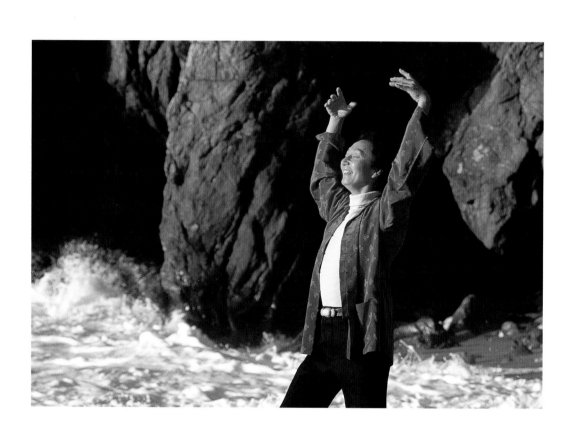

Water

At the completion of Fire, your energy was fully extended, with arms having pushed the Chi forward and upward. Your base was firmly centered between both legs. You are now ready to infuse that power and change it into the gentler Chi of Water. Water is the Yin transformation of the Yang Fire.

Allow the arms to continue to lift high over the crown of your head. Scoop up the energy with your hands and carry it, like a caressing cascade of water downward alongside your face and neck and shoulders and then down into your torso.

Let the rejuvenating quality of this Chi settle and collect back into the receptacle—your Dantien.

Water is to receive

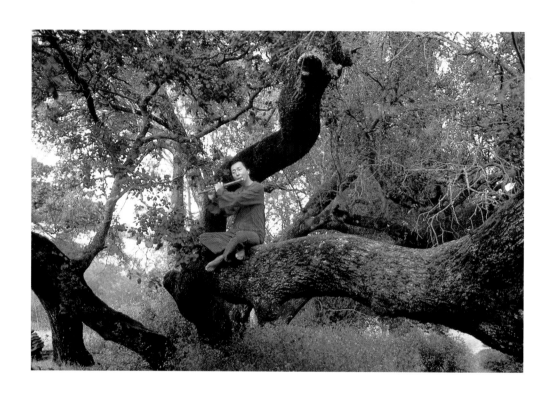

Wood

Tree energy from deep inside the earth begins to germinate, unfurling into roots and trunk, sending out branches, opening into leaves for light and air, and finally bursting into blossoms and fruits. Visualize this growth as you practice this motif.

Continuing from the Water position, visualize your roots stretching down and spreading out all around you.

Slowly walk in a single small circle as your feel your energy unfolding, unwinding.

Let your arms branch out from your torso, extending your Chi and absorbing nourishment.

Survey your panorama. Reach out and touch the world. Enjoy the realization of your full potential as you make your own sweeping orbit within the universe.

Wood is to grow

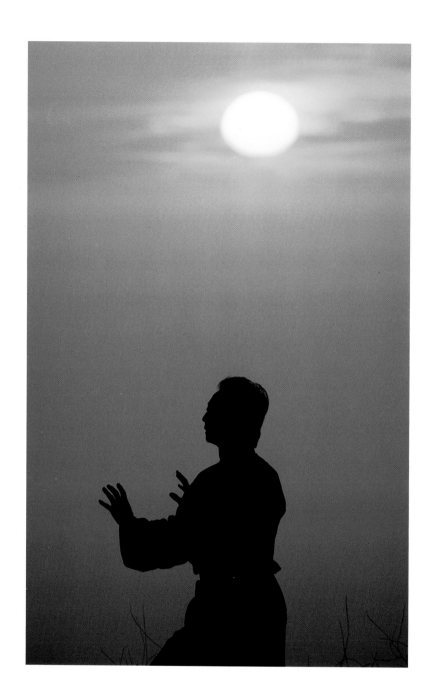

Gold

The growth of Wood must be contained and collected back into the Dantien, the power source. For it is here that we find the cauldron where treasures and metals are alchemized into pure gold.

From the outreaching Wood circle, come back to the basic Tai Ji stance.

With one arm, scoop in with a beckoning gesture all the energy you've created and felt around you.

Lower it, and absorb it into your Dantien.

Repeat with the other arm.

When the energy from both sides has been collected back into your center, focus it into a small, calm crystal, concentrated and with enormous potential.

Gold is to crystalize

Earth

Earth is the mother. We all come from the Earth. We are a part of her organic growth. She is the genesis of all our creative power.

We are going to return Gold back to its Earth source.

Feel the welcoming pull from the earth. Drop your arms and release your holding of the crystal.

Let your arms sweep up to the sky like a funnel. Feel the energy above and the energy below. Become the link, the center between Heaven and Earth.

Now let your arms glide down to settle this new connection into your Dantien.

You have returned to the beginning.

Earth
     is to
          come
               home

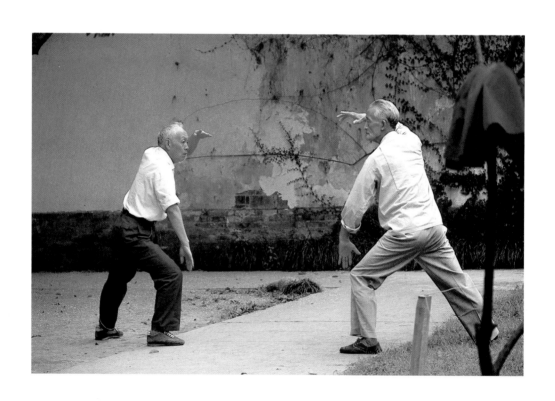

VIII The Practice

Every morning in China, nearly everybody comes out of their house to do some form of Tai Ji exercise in the fresh air. The Chinese believe that a person must begin each day by harmonizing his or her body-mind-spirit with nature.

It would be useless to go to work or enter into daily activities without first becoming awake and energized. Nature provides the unfailing inspiration needed to "get going."

Tai Ji practice need not be obligatory. It can be an enjoyable and self-directed discipline. It becomes a nourishing time for oneself, an important oasis in an otherwise hectic day.

Do not forget that the only Tai Ji tool is the human body, already perfectly attuned to move in the Tai Ji way.

We must learn not to interfere with its organic functioning, but instead, to trust it.

Practice each time like it was the first time. Let your practice be like the sun rising anew every morning.

If you enjoy your practice, you will wish to maintain it, and you will improve.

So an important question becomes, "Do I like it?", not, "Is it good for me?"

Enjoyment of practice means enjoyment of learning.

And most rewarding for me, it means an enjoyment of being a Tai Ji beginner. For Tai Ji is a continuous learning process. One never completes the course, but simply follows the process.

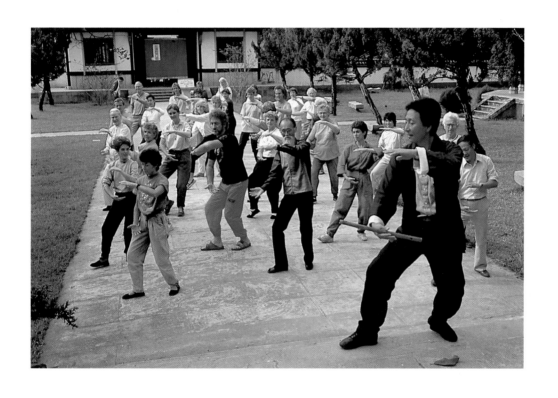

A Tai Ji beginner
is the best student of life,
and for life.

Play your Tai Ji body
like a bamboo flute.
Lift it up to the wind,
it plays itself.
The music comes from
its emptiness.

Don't overwork to
fill yourself with muscles,
ideas and stale information.

A stuffy, rigid body
cannot dance.

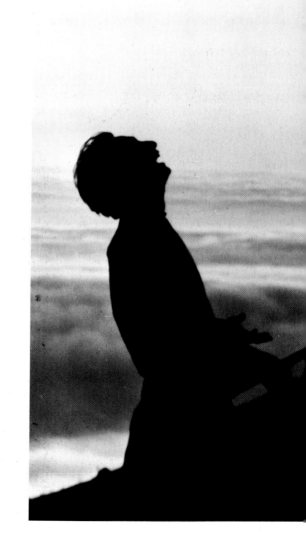

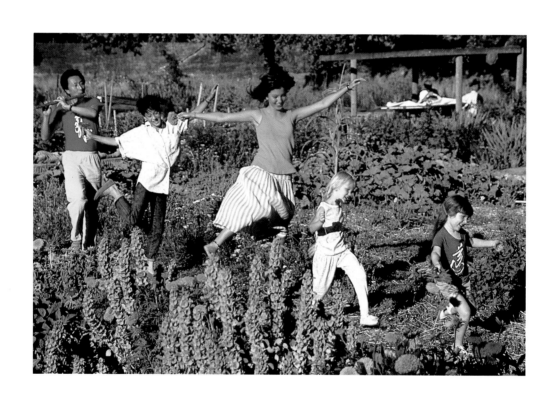

IX Summary

Remember that Tai Ji is natural.

Fish swim and birds fly and humans move—all in the Tai Ji Dance.

The rediscovery of original grace in our daily life is Tai Ji at its most basic and enjoyable.

Our origin is the dance. Our original self is the dancer.

Do not become discouraged at the beginning, as simple and spontaneous things often seem complex and full of effort at first attempt.

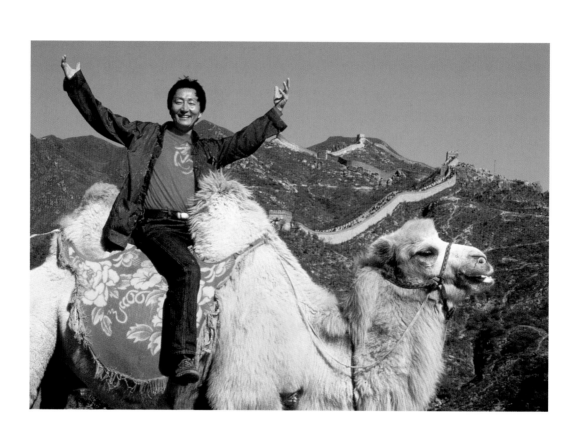

Open your mind. Open your heart. Open your body.

Open your Self.

Relax and smile.

You *are* Tai Ji!

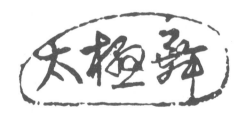

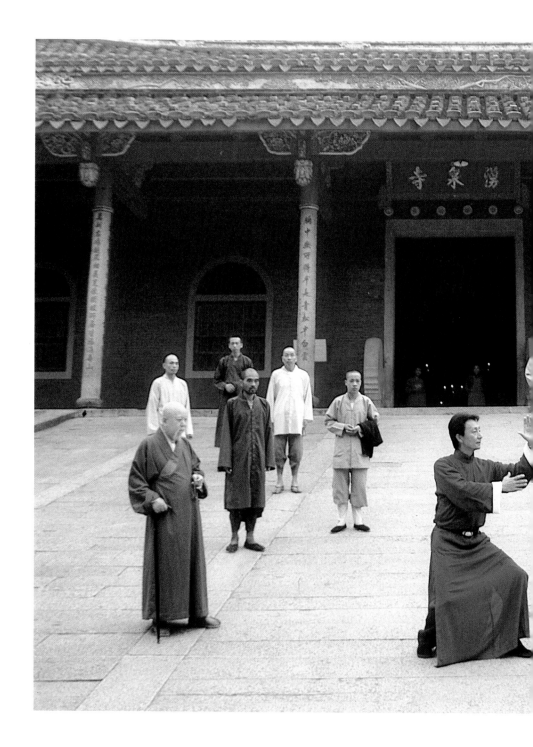

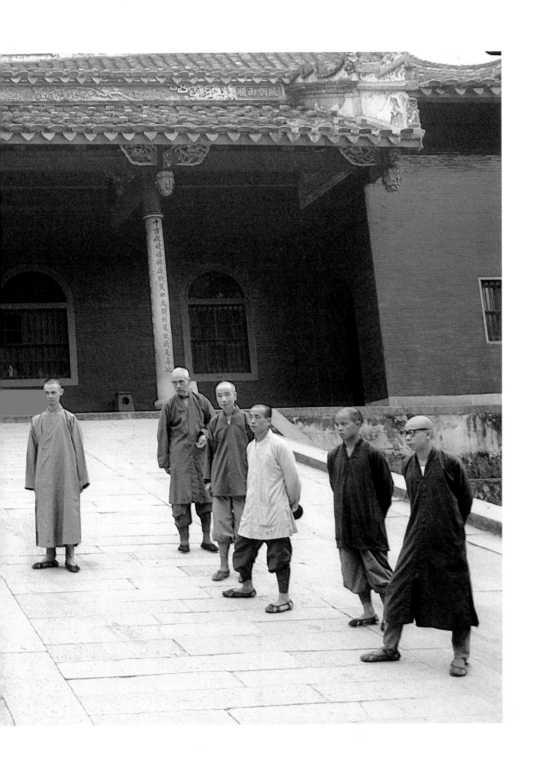

MAN follows the ways of Earth
Earth follows the ways of Heaven
Heaven follows the way of Tao
Tao follows its own nature

Tao Te Ching

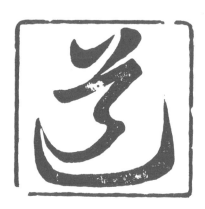

Chungliang Al Huang is President
of the international Living Tao Foundation
and Director of the Lan Ting Institute in
the Sacred Mountains of China and on
the Oregon Coast in America. He is the
author of numerous books, including the
classic, *Embrace Tiger, Return to
Mountain*; *Quantum Soup*; and coauthor
with Alan Watts of *Tao: The Watercourse
Way*; and with Jerry Lynch of *Thinking
Body, Dancing Mind.*

Si Chi Ko is considered a national treasure,
one of the most honored photographers
in China. His work has appeared in pub-
lications and exhibitions throughout the
world. He has collaborated with Master
Huang for over three decades, most
notably in *Embrace Tiger, Return to
Mountain.*

LIVING TAO FOUNDATION

Is a nonprofit organization that is devoted to East/West cultural synthesis, and continues to create unique Tai Ji events—seminars on applying ancient wisdom to modern living throughout the world.
For more information, contact:

LIVING TAO FOUNDATION
P.O. Box 846
Urbana, Illinois 61803-0846
Tel/fax: (217) 337-6113

And by the same author...

EMBRACE TIGER, RETURN TO MOUNTAIN
The Essence of Tai Ji
by Chungliang Al Huang
with photos by Si Chi Ko

The author's unique understanding of eastern tradition, plus his training in dance and martial arts have made him one of the foremost interpreters of Tai Ji and its philosophies. While there are many books currently available on this subject, none have equalled the presentation achieved by EMBRACE TIGER. With a preface by Alan Watts.
$14.95 paper, 256 pages

QUANTUM SOUP
Fortune Cookies in Crisis
by Chungliang Al Huang

This series of philosophical essays links the ancient wisdom of the East with the informality of the West, offering a veritable banquet of food for thought that will set you mind dancing. Lavishly illustrated throughout with the author's own expressive calligraphy—QUANTUM SOUP *is a gourmet preparation of philosophical snips and snails, birds nest, shark's fins and puppy dog's tails to tickle the sophisticated palate and provoke happy, healthful belly laughs. Confucious say: "Number One good recipe!"*
—Joseph Campbell.
$18.95 paper
144 pages

Available from you local bookstore or directly from the publisher. Please include $4.50 shipping and handling for the first book and $1.00 for each additional book. California residents include local sales tax. For more information or our complete catalog of books, posters, and tapes, write to:

CELESTIAL ARTS
P.O. Box 7123
Berkeley, CA 94707

For VISA or MasterCard orders call (800) 841-2665
www.tenspeed.com